Healthy Chocolate!
Too Good To Be True?

Have an Amazing Life
By Eating Chocolate that Is Healthy

A billion people eat chocolate every day! It's an emotional, sensual, mouth-watering comfort food. Most people don't know chocolate is also a nutritious food and one of the healthiest on the planet.

In this sensational Itty Bitty® Book, Dr. Carla, Deeann and Diana reveal how eating healthy chocolate every day can create more happiness, better health and increase longevity.

Discover the 15 compelling facts why chocolate needs to be a daily healthy habit for you and everyone you love.

- Casanova's secret revealed
- Crush the Big C
- Activate your skinny gene
- Banish your blues
- Get more from your workout

If you already love chocolate, pick up a copy of this powerful book today and discover how delicious and beneficial chocolate can really be.

Your Amazing Itty Bitty® Chocolate Book

15 Compelling Facts Why Eating Healthy Chocolate Every Day Can Help You Be Happier, Healthier And Live Longer

Deeann Elder, B.S.
Diana Deene, Ph.D.
Dr. Carla Rudolph, D.C., A.K.

Published by Itty Bitty® Publishing
A subsidiary of S & P Productions, Inc.

Printed in the United States of America

Itty Bitty® Publishing
311 Main Street, Suite D
El Segundo, CA 90245
(310) 640-8885

ISBN: 978-0-9992211-4-3

*The information in this book is not intended or
implied to be a substitute for professional
medical advice, diagnosis or treatment. All
content in this book is for general information
purposes only.*

This book is dedicated to all the chocolate lovers around the world.

This book is also dedicated to everyone interested in enjoying a nutritious diet and a healthy life.

A special thank you to Shirlee and Art Martinez, Susan Rothwell, Andy and Shari Rosenberg, Gale Wong, Lisa Poliak, John Dade and Jeremy Elder for their support and contributions.

Stop by our Itty Bitty® website to find interesting information regarding health-enhancing chocolate.

www.IttyBittyPublishing.com

Or visit us at

IttyBittyChocolateBook.com

Table of Contents

Introduction

If you love chocolate, or even just like it, you owe it to yourself to read this book. You'll learn some surprising truths about this important food.

It's not just candy! It's not just dark chocolate! It's not just a sinful indulgence we crave and try to avoid.

You can't be blamed for being skeptical. There is a long-standing belief that chocolate is not good for you. So how can it be healthy?

The truth is – pure unadulterated chocolate is one of the healthiest foods you can eat. And your body has an innate ability to stay healthy or heal when given the proper nutrition and tools. In this book the words chocolate, cacao and cocoa refer to the same delicious, mood enhancing and health-promoting food.

Chocolate is a mouth-watering, emotional, sensual, delicious food that can help you be healthier, be happier and slow the aging process. In fact, chocolate is often considered nature's perfect food. Hard to believe? Yet, it's true. Chocolate comes from the cocoa bean and that bean is a nutritional powerhouse.

The ancient peoples of Central America knew the nutritional power of cocoa thousands of years ago without any support from scientific evidence. The

Aztec and Mayan cultures drank a bitter cocoa beverage for nourishment, energy and medicinal purposes. The cocoa bean was so valuable it was used in worship and as money.

The ancient Aztec emperor Montezuma was one of the original chocoholics. He was known to drink fifty cups of chocolate a day.

Today, with so much information available about chocolate, it is easy to be confused. We are bombarded with many mixed messages from the media, advertisers and doctors.

This Itty Bitty® Book draws upon evidence-based results from thousands of independent scientific studies conducted at prestigious institutions during the last 15 to 20 years. Much of the research uses unprocessed, non-alkalized cocoa powder. These results confirm the multitude of health benefits dark chocolate provides. Your beliefs about chocolate may be challenged and require a paradigm shift.

After reading <u>Your Amazing Itty Bitty®</u> <u>Chocolate Book</u>, we hope you'll be inspired enough by some of the evidence-based truths about chocolate and instead of saying, *"I can't eat chocolate,"* you'll start saying, *"Wow! I must eat chocolate every day."*

Fact 1
Chocolate Is The World's Favorite Food

If you're like the average person, you eat about 12 pounds of chocolate every year. The problem is most people are eating unhealthy chocolate, stripped of its numerous nutrients. For thousands of years chocolate was considered a miraculous food and one of nature's original health foods. After chocolate was introduced to Europe in the 1500s, it became a confection and the health benefits began to vanish. In recent history, science has rediscovered the abundant health benefits in pure chocolate. These health benefits, along with the delicious taste, are good reasons to continue your love affair with chocolate, guilt-free. It's not just a sinful indulgence.

1. Chocolate symbolizes, as does no other food, luxury, comfort, sensuality, gratification and love.
2. 52% of Americans claim chocolate is their favorite flavor.
3. Global chocolate sales exceed ninety-five billion dollars annually.
4. Many exploding scientific studies about health have focused on chocolate for its promising health benefits. These benefits seem to increase every year.

What People Are Saying About Chocolate

"The superiority of chocolate for health and nourishment will soon give it the same preference over tea and coffee in America as it has in Spain."

Thomas Jefferson

- German biochemist Baron von Liebig (1800s) said, *"Chocolate is a perfect food – as wholesome as it is delicious, a beneficent restorer of exhausted power, but its quality must be good and it must be carefully prepared."*
- Put 'eat chocolate' at the top of your list of things to do today and at least you'll get one thing done.
- Chocolate is a delicious cure for a bad day.
- A little too much chocolate is just about right.
- When life gives you lemons, throw them back and ask for chocolate.
- The 12-Step Chocoholics Program: Never be more than 12-steps away from chocolate.
- Chocolate comes from cocoa which is a tree. That makes it a plant. Therefore, chocolate is a salad.
- We must all believe in something. I believe I'll have another piece of healthy chocolate.

Fact 2
SURPRISE!
Chocolate Can Be Good For You

You probably have heard chocolate, not chocolate candy, is good for you. Scientific methods are now sophisticated enough to better analyze the nutritional content of foods. In fact, scientists were surprised to discover chocolate's impressive nutritional profile and health benefits.

1. Surprisingly, chocolate is rich in a variety of nutrients that give it energy-boosting, disease-preventing properties that rival the nutritional power of many commonplace fruits and vegetables.
2. Chocolate in its natural state has numerous vitamins, minerals, amino acids, carbohydrates, healthy fats, enzymes and an extremely high amount of antioxidants, flavonoids and polyphenols.
3. Eating healthy, dark chocolate daily is a delicious way to nourish your body and support your health. In the following chapters, we provide evidence that the consumption of cocoa can lower the risk of cancer, support heart health, reduce chronic inflammation and protect the brain – to name a few.

Chocolate Is One Of The World's Healthiest Foods

"The cocoa bean is a phenomenon, for nowhere else has nature concentrated such a wealth of valuable nourishment in so small a space."
Alexander von Humboldt
(1800s German Scientist)

- Surprisingly, the cocoa bean contains more than 150 essential nutrients.
- Unprocessed chocolate is the highest natural source of iron in food.
- Chocolate is one of the highest sources of magnesium, which is one of the most important minerals in our diet. It is also one in which people are the most deficient.
- Some other minerals in chocolate include calcium, zinc, copper and phosphorus.
- Vitamins B, C and E are just a few of the essential nutrients found in chocolate.
- *"Healthy chocolate; it sounded too good to be true. However, I investigated the products thoroughly ... I soon experienced the benefits of this amazing product and saw positive results in my patients."* Dr. Alan W. Gruning, D.O., Florida
- Given the research, never underestimate the power of chocolate.

Fact 3
Chocolate Is Your Weight-Loss Friend

According to Jackie Gleason, *"The second day of a diet is always easier than the first. By the second day you're off it."* This may not be accurate, but the fact that roughly 108 million American dieters typically make four to five attempts per year certainly underscores the difficulty most of us have staying on a weight-loss program. Obesity and just being overweight have become health problems of epidemic proportions with serious associated health risks such as heart disease, diabetes, cancer and arthritis.

1. Studies show the flavonoids in healthy chocolate can stimulate the Sirt-1 gene, often called your "skinny gene," which assists with weight loss by inhibiting fat storage and increasing fat metabolism.
2. Chocolate's theobromine has some unique fat-loss properties. It helps control and suppress appetite and moves fatty acids from fat cells to the blood stream where they are burned as energy.
3. Dark chocolate helps sustain a healthy weight by stabilizing blood-sugar, reducing inflammation and fat storage, restoring digestive function, controlling appetite and curbing cravings.

Eat Chocolate To Lose And Maintain Your Weight Goals

- Many health professionals now recommend chocolate as part of a healthy wellness regimen to lose weight, stay on your program and maintain your desired weight.
- According to a Queen Margaret University study, *"Dark chocolate has an impressive impact on how the body synthesizes fatty acids, thus reducing the digestion and absorption of fats and carbohydrates."*
- Chocolate's antioxidants can normalize cell receptor-site sensitivity and enzyme activity, resulting in less fluid retention and fat accumulation.
- The cocoa butter in chocolate has many essential fats that are good for you and also aids in shedding unwanted pounds and inches.
- A twelve-week study on chocolate and weight-loss using a high-antioxidant chocolate meal replacement shake resulted in an average weight loss of 31.3 pounds and an average waist circumference decrease of 5.8 inches. Published in Am. Jr. of Bariatric Med.
- Julie in Wisconsin shed 58 pounds in 5 months and reduced snacking by eating 3 pieces of high-antioxidant chocolate and replacing her evening meal with the high-antioxidant chocolate shake daily.

Fact 4
Chocolate Fights Cancer

Cancer, in its many forms, is on the rise and is one of the most feared and pervasive diseases. Most of us have at least one friend or family member who has been treated for some type of cancer. While progress has been made in the treatment of many cancers, there is still much to be learned. Fortunately, scientific studies have revealed the potential of chocolate's primary compounds to help protect cells and fight cancer.

1. A 2005 study at Georgetown University Medical Center treated the four proteins that contribute to the division and growth of breast cancer cells with a procyanidin compound, one of chocolate's numerous antioxidants. All four were essentially "turned off," and the cancer cells stopped dividing.
2. Chocolate may reduce cancer risk by stimulating the production of tumor necrosis factor (TNF), a protein that preferentially targets tumors.
3. Chocolate's antioxidants can prevent cancer by preserving normal cell regulation. This helps keep cells healthy and stops damage to DNA, which can contribute to development of cancers.

Chocolate Can Inhibit Cancer

- According to the National Foundation for Cancer Research, dark chocolate contains powerful cancer-fighting antioxidants.
- A study at Harvard University led by Dr. Norman Hollenberg, M.D., compared rates of cancer and heart disease in Panama's island-dwelling Kuna Indians who drink an average of 5 cups of cocoa daily to mainland-living Kuna who don't. Islanders' rates of these two diseases are far lower than those of the mainlanders and most other populations.
- Chocolate decreases inflammation, a key contributor to cancer formation.
- Decreasing inflammation stops cell proliferation and aids the apoptosis (death) of cancer cells.
- Chocolate's antioxidants stimulate the activities of detoxification enzymes and help minimize damage to DNA.
- Antioxidants can help prevent tumors from invading normal tissue by decreasing certain enzymes that contribute to tumor growth.

Fact 5
Chocolate Boosts Passion
And Enhances Well-Being

We all know we eat chocolate because it tastes so good and it also makes us feel so good. This sense of happiness and pleasure, often called the bliss factor, is the reason nine out of ten people love chocolate and five out of ten crave it.

1. The compounds in chocolate trigger the release of mood-enhancing chemicals in the brain, which can optimize mood, emotional health and a sense of euphoria.
2. The "love chemical" PEA (phenylethylamine), which is found in chocolate, stimulates a sense of well-being, pleasure and contentment.
3. The "bliss" chemical, anandamide, also found in chocolate, promotes and maintains feelings of well-being.
4. Eating chocolate helps release the "cuddle" hormone, oxytocin, and can increase your ability to feel closer.
5. Cocoa contains significant amounts of the amino acid tryptophan. Tryptophan increases levels of dopamine and serotonin, which are natural antidepressants and also can help you relax and sleep better.

Chocolate Naturally Enhances Your Passion And Well-Being

- Chocolate has an antidepressant effect because of its ability to increase neurotransmitters, elevate mood and help decrease the "Monday Morning Blues."
- Casanova often ate chocolate because of its aphrodisiac properties.
- People express their love of chocolate by saying things like: *"Sadness is no chocolate in the house,"* or *"Chocolate is cheaper than therapy and you don't need an appointment."*
- *"A friend of mine once said, 'Life is meant to be enjoyed, not endured!' Thanks to healthy chocolate, I am back to enjoying life again no matter what negative comment or situation comes my way."* Scott K. Tennessee

Fact 6
Antioxidants Are Important

Antioxidants neutralize the damaging effects of
free radicals and toxins. Oxidative cell damage
is caused by free radicals and occurs when we
breathe, eat, sleep and move. Oxidation rots
fruit, fades paint, rusts metal and ages people.
Your body produces some antioxidants, but not
as many as people need, given our complex
lifestyles and toxic environments. Additionally,
it's important to know that oxidative damage is
linked to more than 200 chronic diseases,
including the big four: cancer, heart disease,
diabetes and stroke.

1. At least 10,000 free radicals attack our
   cells hourly. Experts advise eating at
   least 100,000 antioxidants daily to help
   protect against free radical damage.
2. Antioxidants should be replenished at
   least every four to five hours because
   your body does not store them.
3. We are told to eat 8 to 10 servings of
   fruits and vegetables daily because
   they're antioxidant foods.
4. Chocolate is one of the best sources of
   antioxidants and eating small amounts of
   chocolate can provide huge benefits.

Antioxidant-Rich Foods

Antioxidants are often measured and reported as an ORAC (Oxygen Radical Absorbance Capacity) score.

Antioxidant Values of Common Foods

Food	ORAC per 100g (3.5 oz)
Cold pressed Cocoa Powder	34,396
Acai Berry	18,500
Dark Chocolate	13,120
Milk Chocolate	6,740
Prunes	5,770
Red Wine	3,524
Pomegranate	3,307
Blueberries	2,400
Blackberries	2,035
Kale	1,770
Cranberries	1,750
Strawberries	1,540
Spinach	1,260
Raspberries	1,220
Brussels Sprouts	980
Plums	949
Alfalfa Sprouts	930
Broccoli Florets	890
Beets	840
Oranges	750
Red Grapes	739
Red Bell Pepper	710
Cherries	670

Fact 7
Chocolate Is An Antioxidant Wonder

Today science has rediscovered what the ancient civilizations knew: chocolate is good for you. Its high antioxidant content provides many of the health benefits science is now uncovering.

1. For centuries, civilizations used chocolate medicinally without knowing any of the scientific reasons.
2. Hernán Cortéz, who introduced chocolate to Europe in the 16th Century, said, *"A cup of this precious drink permits a man to walk for a whole day without food."*
3. According to an article in the Journal of Nutrition, chocolate was historically used to treat many conditions including cough, colds, cancer, inflammation, menstrual flow and obesity.
4. To date, thousands of articles have focused on chocolate and human health. Many of the health benefits are attributed to chocolate's antioxidant content.
5. Cocoa beans are super-rich in antioxidant flavonols. According to research cited in The New York Times one hundred grams of cocoa beans contain 10 grams of flavonol antioxidants, which makes cocoa one of the richest sources of antioxidants of any food.

Chocolate Is A Potent Antioxidant Food

- Darker is better. Antioxidants contribute to chocolate's color. The more flavonoids, the darker the chocolate and potentially the greater the health benefits.
- Dark chocolate has numerous different antioxidants, which act synergistically to amplify each other and magnify the antioxidant benefits.
- Dr. Chang Y. Le, M.D., of Cornell University, found that chocolate is a great source of antioxidants because it has more antioxidants than a glass of red wine or a cup of green tea.
- *"The antioxidants found in chocolate are among the most important observations in the history of medicine."* Dr. Norman Hollenberg, M.D., Harvard University
- Science continues to discover multiple benefits derived from daily consumption of chocolate, even though the amazing chemistry in the fruit and seeds of the tropical cocoa tree remains mysterious.
- Cocoa's antioxidants are very stable and easily available to human metabolism.
- White chocolate contains no cocoa solids, so it is not a good source of antioxidants. University of Michigan
- When looking for a high antioxidant food healthy chocolate is the best choice.

Fact 8
Chocolate Promotes Longevity

Aging is a progressive deterioration of the body that causes wrinkles, aching muscles and joints, diminished energy levels and much more. When healthy, the body staves off deterioration through cell reproduction and renewal. Protecting cells and their reproductive ability is key to increasing longevity and vitality. Again, research indicates antioxidants are a compelling defense against free radical cellular damage and its associated effects on aging.

1. According to science, aging happens as the normal maintenance and repair systems in the body weaken over time. The pace at which cells break down, or age, can be greatly influenced by how well we nourish them.

2. Chocolate contains resveratrol. Resveratrol is one of the only substances known to science that seems to directly extend lifespan by helping to activate the Sirt-1, or longevity, gene. (Sirt-1 is also your skinny gene as stated in Fact 3.)

3. Chocolate's antioxidants can protect telomeres (the parts of chromosomes that control aging, safeguard DNA and influence cell reproduction) from free radical damage.

Stay Young With Chocolate

- Cells constantly replace themselves with new copies. Healthy telomeres prevent small errors in this replication process.
- The antioxidants and phytonutrients in chocolate protect cells and DNA from damage and mutation.
- Chocolate's antioxidants help protect the skin from UV light and the damage it causes.
- Chocolate's nutritional powerhouse and antioxidants can help repair damaged cells so they don't continue down their destructive path, which can lead to life-threatening diseases.
- *"The persons who habitually take chocolate are those who enjoy the most equable and constant health and are least liable to a multitude of illnesses which spoil the enjoyment of life."* A. Brillat-Savarin, 18th Century Gastronome and Epicure
- *"Daily use of antioxidants can add 10 healthful years to your life."* UCLA Medical School
- *"I'm 92 years old and have been eating healthy chocolate since 2007. I live independently, work in my yard and drive. I was even able to dance at my 90th birthday party."* Eleanor S., Indiana

Fact 9
Chocolate Supports Immune Function & Defends Against Chronic Inflammation

The immune system is designed to protect your body against the millions of bacteria, viruses, toxins, parasites and microbes that can compromise it. A compromised immune system can make you sick and can cause inflammatory and autoimmune diseases.

1. Chronic inflammation is insidious, silent, and quite dangerous. Because it is painless, it can go unrecognized for years, and can wear down your body.
2. Studies have shown that a cocoa enriched diet improves T-cell function and increases your gut's antibodies, thus boosting your immune system's defenses.
3. Scientists agree that one benefit of healthy dark chocolate is its ability to prevent or even reverse damaging chronic inflammation.
4. *"Chronic health conditions begin with low-grade inflammation. Everything from cardiovascular disease to diabetes begins with specific tissue damage caused by ... inflammation. Healthy chocolate prevents ... inflammation and tissue damage."* Dr. B. Phillips, D.C., Indiana

17

Chocolate Supports Immune Function And Relieves Inflammation

- The inflammatory response in your body results from free radical damage to cells, tissues and organs. The high antioxidants in chocolate reduce inflammation.
- Chocolate's cell-signaling system supports cellular communication and improves immune responses.
- Chronic inflammation is the underlying cause of heart disease, cancer and many other chronic diseases.
- University of Southampton researchers said inflammation in the brain is what drives Alzheimer's disease.
- Chocolate as an immune controller may have therapeutic benefits in diseases that involve overstimulation of the immune system, including eczema and arthritis.
- Results from one study on chronic fatigue syndrome found that the variety of chocolate's chemicals provide an energy lift, decrease anxiety and reduce pain and inflammation.
- *"I had Systemic Lupus, an auto-immune disease, for 12-years. I'm happy to say consuming healthy chocolate daily completely changed my life. I am now off five medications and feel better than I have in 12-years."* Dana A., Indiana

Fact 10
Chocolate Keeps Your Heart Healthy

Heart disease is the number-one killer in the United States and many European countries. Someone in the US dies from cardiovascular disease every 33 seconds. Heart health has been the focus of more chocolate research than any other disease or area of health.

1. Cardiovascular diseases are disorders that affect the function of the heart and blood vessels. Common forms of heart disease are high blood pressure, congestive heart failure, atherosclerosis, stroke and coronary artery disease.
2. Damage to the lining of blood vessel walls is a major factor in cardiovascular disease, heart attack, stroke and other coronary events.
3. Chocolate enhances the availability of nitric oxide, which declines as we age.
4. Nitric oxide is important to a healthy heart because it widens veins and arteries, improves blood flow and strengthens cardiac function.
5. Additionally, nitric oxide is important for many organ systems, including sexual function.

Chocolate Supports Heart Health

- *"Chocolate can potentially support overall cardiovascular health."* Eliot Brinton, M.D. University of Utah
- Howard LeWine, M.D., wrote in Harvard Health Publications, *"If you're a chocoholic, the news out of England is tantalizing: middle-aged and older adults who eat up to 3.5 ounces of chocolate a day seem to have lower rates of heart disease than those who spurn chocolate."*
- Chocolate decreases blood clotting, thereby reducing the risk of stroke.
- Chocolate may improve blood pressure and decrease blood vessel inflammation.
- Studies on chocolate and heart disease found that people who consumed an average of six grams of dark chocolate a day had about a 40% lower chance of suffering a heart attack or stroke.
- Chocolate increases levels of HDL, the good cholesterol, and lowers levels of LDL, the bad cholesterol.
- Researchers found that stearic acid, the principal fat in unprocessed chocolate, does not have adverse cardiovascular health effects. It is metabolized differently than other saturated fats.

Fact 11
Chocolate Protects Your Brain

Recent surveys show Americans fear developing Alzheimer's and dementia more than any other life-threatening disease, even cancer. Free radical damage can affect your brain's health and its cognitive abilities. Chocolate's rich antioxidants have the ability to protect your brain from neurodegenerative diseases. Think about it, it's never too soon to start caring for your brain.

1. Great news! Antioxidants in healthy chocolate protect the brain from aging wear and tear, can defend the brain from conditions related to high blood pressure and clots and can help reverse brain damage and restore brain function.
2. British scientists determined that chocolate could slow the buildup of amyloid plaque, reducing the likelihood of Alzheimer's and other dementia.
3. A Columbia University study found chocolate's antioxidants reversed memory decline in healthy older adults.
4. A Harvard study found chocolate consumption boosts thinking and memory performance. Chocolate's antioxidants increase blood flow in the brain, allowing more blood, oxygen and other nutrients to reach key areas.

Boosting and Protecting Brain Health

- Anandamide, a chemical in chocolate, supports brain health and could be helpful for multiple sclerosis patients.
- *"Having MS, I experienced multiple symptoms and took medications for each one. I could barely walk. Healthy chocolate daily gave me a quality of life I would never have known without it. All of my lesions are inactive and I only need my MS injection. I pursue most activities that interest me and have even learned to Elk & Deer hunt."* Norma S., Nevada
- Chocolate's antioxidant, cell-signaling and anti-inflammatory mechanisms could improve Parkinson's symptoms. Dresden University of Technology
- *"Living with Parkinson's is not easy. I had to stop to rest at least twice when covering the 200 feet from my house to my barn. I stopped restoring antique tractors. I was introduced to healthy chocolate and began to notice changes: more energy, less pain. Now, with healthy chocolate I'm able to work on my tractors, mow the lawn and plant a garden. Oh, yes, I now jog to the barn."* David R., Tennessee
- Research has also shown that chocolate can benefit people with ADD and ADHD by improving focus.

Fact 12
Chocolate Helps Diabetics Stay Healthy

Diabetes is one of the most promising areas in which chocolate supports better health. Poor diet and out-of-balance blood-sugar levels contribute to the explosion of obesity, type-2 diabetes and other related conditions. Chocolate's antioxidants can protect against the effects of diabetes.

1. Chocolate's antioxidants can improve the utilization of insulin in diabetic patients by making the body more insulin sensitive to decrease blood-sugar levels.
2. Elevated blood-sugar levels can cause micro blood vessel damage and can result in blood vessel blockage, neuropathy and edema, ultimately leading to ulcerations and amputations.
3. Chocolate helps prevent blood vessel damage by stimulating the production of nitric oxide, which improves blood flow in veins and arteries.
4. *"As a medical doctor, I want to improve people's health. ... I recommend healthy chocolate as a health supplement in my medical practice when transitioning people to a healthier lifestyle. My patients have experienced improvements in weight loss, blood pressure and diabetes."* Dr. Alicia A., M.D., Tenn.

Healthy Chocolate Is Diabetic Friendly

- It's best for diabetics to choose cold-pressed chocolate because of its high-antioxidant content and its ability to help maintain a low glycemic index.
- Chocolate's antioxidants improve insulin sensitivity because of their ability to fight free radicals, increase the availability of nitric oxide and reduce inflammation at the cellular level.
- Chocolate can protect blood vessels from scarring. Blood vessel scarring can cause kidney damage and even blindness.
- Chocolate reduces cardiovascular symptoms related to blood-glucose irregularities by balancing blood-sugar levels.
- *"Emerging research suggests that damage to the cells' mitochondria, which occurs from repeated "attacks" by free radicals, contributes to the nerve pain (neuropathy) common to diabetics. Taken in context, it is feasible that cocoa's powerful antioxidant capabilities could then prevent or relieve the nerve pain so many diabetics suffer from."* Lisa Getas, D.C. Nevada

Fact 13
Chocolate Enhances Your Workout

When you exercise, an added measure of nutrition may be needed for more energy and faster recovery. Additionally, free radical damage increases as you increase your physical activity. Antioxidants are needed to neutralize free radical damage. Therefore active people must eat high-antioxidant dark chocolate every day.

1. Chocolate is emerging as a delicious, nutrient-rich food for increasing your physical performance.
2. Flavonoid-rich dark chocolate increases heart rates and oxygen consumption. In a Kingston University study, dark chocolate-snacking bicyclists used less oxygen and covered a greater distance in a two-minute timed trial than white chocolate-snacking cyclists.
3. In the same study, chocolate's antioxidants increased nitric oxide production in the body, which helps boost endurance and strength.
4. Chocolate offers an unexpected way to enhance your workout. Chocolate's exercise-improvement arsenal includes energy-rich nutrients, antioxidant-repair mechanisms and protection of the heart and vascular systems.

Chocolate Helps You Exercise Better

- Healthy chocolate boosts energy safely, effectively and naturally because it increases blood flow.
- A new study shows you can perform better if you eat dark chocolate just before your workout. Flavonoids in dark chocolate bind to receptors in muscles, which helps them resist fatigue.
- Chocolate's distinct anti-inflammatory properties accelerate recovery and reduce the soreness and pain associated with athletic activity.
- Chocolate can help repair exercise-induced muscle damage and enhance energy metabolism.
- Chocolate helps reduce the Monday morning aches and pains that weekend warriors often experience.
- *"I am active duty military and have always been an athletic individual . . . I consider myself to be athletic and participated in an Ironman triathlon. I began incorporating healthy chocolate into my nutritional plan and found myself recovering faster and getting stronger. Without healthy chocolate, I would not have been able to successfully complete the race."* Rob K., Illinois
- Be good to yourself and eat healthy chocolate when working out.

Fact 14
The Way Chocolate Is Processed Is Extremely Important

Historically, chocolate has been an amazing food to support health. Manufacturing methods during the last 200 years have often changed nutritious chocolate into nutritionally empty candy. Therefore, it is imperative to distinguish between healthy chocolate and chocolate candy.

1. The Cleveland Clinic wisely points out, *"Most commercial (candy) chocolates are highly processed. The more chocolate is processed (through things like fermentation, alkalizing, roasting, etc.), the more antioxidants are lost."*
2. To prevent degradation of cocoa's antioxidants and beneficial nutrients, it is best to process cocoa at temperatures at or below 110°F. Cold-pressed cocoa maintains considerably more antioxidants than roasted and heated cocoa.
3. Manufacturing of chocolate when making candy usually destroys most of chocolate's beneficial nutrients and antioxidants. Cocoa beans are roasted (up to 266°F) and refined sugars are added.
4. Often alkali is added to cocoa when manufacturing chocolate further destroying its antioxidants and nutrients.

Know Your Chocolate!

- Chocolate should be at least 70% cocoa.
- The National Chocolate Council says, *"The percentage of cacao may not indicate a chocolate's health and anti-aging benefits. How the cocoa bean is processed is more important than the percentage of chocolate when determining health benefits."*
- Cold-pressed chocolate retains the greatest amounts of health-enhancing antioxidants and nutrients.
- A healthy chocolate should have its natural cocoa butters and cocoa solids intact as primary ingredients – no hydrogenated oils or fats. Remember, cocoa butter is a healthy, beneficial fat.
- Most chocolate candy sold today should be avoided, as it generally contains over 51% sugars, fats, waxes, oils and preservatives, thereby making chocolate candy just another high calorie, flavorful-yet-toxic delicacy.
- In the early 1800s, manufacturers began adding milk to chocolate, unknowingly compromising cocoa's antioxidants.
- *"Milk chocolate is not a good source of antioxidants because the milk binds to the antioxidants and makes them unavailable."* The University of Michigan

Fact 15
How To Find Healthy Chocolate

Eating healthy, mouthwatering dark chocolate daily is an important lifestyle choice. Unfortunately, not all chocolate is created equal. Take responsibility for your chocolate choices. Cold-pressed chocolate delivers a high amount of antioxidants and nutrients, unlike chocolate candy. It's a healthy and delicious choice. Look for the following on the label. If it's missing, call the company or peruse their website.

1. Read labels! Chocolate is only as good for you as its ingredients. Chocolate or cocoa should be the first ingredient listed.
2. Most people think 70% cocoa is a healthy chocolate. The fact is the amount of antioxidants the chocolate delivers provides the health benefits regardless of the percentage of cocoa. Look for the amount of antioxidants, not the percentage of cocoa on the label.
3. Even though expensive, a few companies know the importance of antioxidants, so they test, measure and list the amount of antioxidants on the label.
4. It is best to look for natural cocoa butter and minimal amounts of sugar.
5. Avoid alkali and 'fillers' such as milk solids, oils or artificial preservatives.

Choose Healthy Chocolate

- This book is designed to help you understand the antioxidant and nutritional benefits provided by eating a high-antioxidant, healthy chocolate every day.
- *"The Beverage of the gods was Ambrosia; that of man is chocolate. Both increase the length of life in a prodigious manner."* Louis Lewin, M.D. (19th century German pharmacologist)
- Many health-care professionals know healthy chocolate is an antioxidant powerhouse. It is one of the world's healthiest foods and they recommend incorporating it into your daily diet.
- People all over the world are discovering chocolate's health benefits and replacing their chocolate candy with delicious healthy chocolate.
- One of the best reasons to choose healthy chocolate is summed up by Dr. Richard Cutler, M.D. NIH. *"The amount of antioxidants that you maintain in your body is directly proportional to how long and healthy you will live."*
- **Your chocolate choice can be life-changing. Now that you understand the importance of antioxidants, stop saying, *"I can't eat chocolate"* and start saying *"I must eat high-antioxidant, healthy chocolate every day."***

You've finished. Before you go...

<u>Tweet/share that you finished this book.</u>

Please star rate this book.

Reviews are solid gold to writers. Please take a few minutes to give us some itty bitty feedback.

ABOUT THE AUTHORS

Deeann Elder is passionate about people and their
health. Her friends call her their personal
cheerleader, as she is always in their corner. For
many years she has been interested in nutrition
and taught classes at Orange Coast College,
including a course on Modern Meals. Her thirst
for knowledge leads her to continually learn and
implement that information in daily life. Deeann
is an enthusiastic reader and loves to travel,
especially taking leisurely road trips. Deeann
graduated with honors, earning a Bachelor of
Science Degree in Home Economics at CSULB.

Diana Deene's strong desire to help people live
happier, more fulfilling lives, led her to spend
more than 30 years as a psychotherapist. She has
long been on the forefront of innovations in
holistic health, focusing on nutrition and
practicing yoga long before there was a yoga
studio on every corner. Diana delights in playing
brain games, reading fiction, attending live
theater and exploring her creativity. She earned
her Bachelor of Arts Degree in Psychology at
Mills College and her doctorate at the California
School of Professional Psychology.

Dr. Carla Rudolph is a holistic healthcare
practitioner whose patients often call her an
architect of modern-day health care. With more
than 25 years of chiropractic experience, Dr.
Carla has always been on the forefront of
advanced health care and loves discovering new
approaches to wellness and longevity. Her

expertise in alternative and complementary medicine, as well as her education and experience in applied kinesiology and nutritional counseling, have led her to specialize in working with and solving difficult cases. Dr. Rudolph earned her BA degree with honors at UC Davis, graduated with honors from Palmer West Chiropractic College, and completed post-graduate studies at Western States Chiropractic College.

Deeann, Diana and Dr. Carla met several years ago, drawn to a seminar on the health benefits of chocolate. All three share an interest in nutrition, health and wellness. They believe a personalized path to preventative care and wellness is extremely important in helping people achieve their health goals. They came together, realizing there was a need to share their combined knowledge that indeed chocolate can be healthy.

Visit www.ittybittychocolatebook.com for additional information, recommendations and updates about Healthy Chocolate

If you liked this Amazing Itty Bitty® Book you might also enjoy…

- **Your Amazing Itty Bitty® Imagery Book** - Rhonda Jordan

- **Your Amazing Itty Bitty® Heal Your Body Book** – Patricia Garza Pinto

- **Your Amazing Itty Bitty® Veterans Survival Book** - Earl J. Katigbak

And many of our other Itty Bitty® books available on line.

www.ingramcontent.com/pod-product-compliance
Lightning Source LLC
Chambersburg PA
CBHW060658280326
41933CB00012B/2235